Organic Recipes for Perfect Skin:
Homemade Recipes of Body Butters, Lotions, Balms, Bath Bombs, and Scrubs that Make Skin Unbelievably Smooth!

Table of content

Introduction

I wish to thank and congratulate you for downloading *"Organic Recipes for Perfect Skin: Homemade Recipes of Body Butters, Lotions, Balms, Bath Bombs that Make Skin Unbelievably Smooth!"* Using this collection of natural homemade products is going to do wonders for the health of your skin. You will see positive results in no time, being able to see and feel the difference in the improved look and overall health of your skin.

Using natural homemade products for your skin will have you feeling and looking better than you have in a long time. They will certainly be a much wiser choice in skin products over using synthetic skin products that have all kinds of chemicals and additives in them that can be harmful to your health and well-being.

More and more people are looking towards choosing natural products for different areas in their lives, including the care of their skin. When you have great looking skin, you are naturally going to feel happier and better about yourself, this will give you a boost that will be like a natural high! Just follow these easy to prepare recipes and you will have that healthy skin you have been wanting in no time at all!

Chapter 1. Anatomy of Our Skin

The human skin is made up of three layers: Epidermis, Dermis, and Subcutaneous fat.

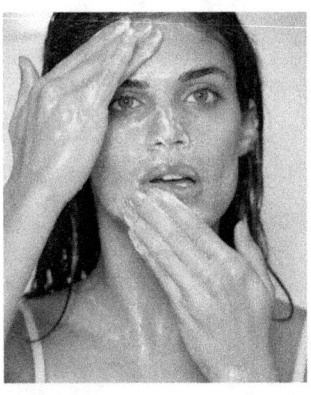

Epidermis: The epidermis is the outer layer of human skin. This is the layer of skin that is visible to the naked eye. This is the part of our skin that all can see, including any imperfections on it such as wrinkles and dry flaky skin. Just below this layer is a very busy network of cells and tissues working hard to produce new cells. In about a two-week period, the new cells will make their way up towards the epidermis. The cells that are already on the epidermis will die and eventually shed off, thereby making room for the new cells. It is quite amazing, but we shed approximately 35,000 old cells every minute.

Just think that while you are reading this you have shed about 70,000 old skin cells! Is that not mind-blowing? So, you can see that your epidermis is hard at work in creating new skin cells for you. It will spend about 95% of its time creating new skin cells. The other 5% percent of its time is spent producing melanin—this is the pigment that adds color to your skin.

Dermis: The dermis is the layer of skin that lies just below the epidermis. This is the area of the human where sweat glands, oil glands, blood vessels, and nerves are located. You may have heard of fibers termed as collagen and elastic, this is the are of the skin where you will find them. The nerve endings are found in this area, providing you with sensations of cold, heat, pain etc. Blood vessels are in the dermis that supply the body with oxygen and nutrients. The oil glands in the skin are also referred to as sebaceous glands, helping with the production of the skin's natural oil called sebum. This helps to lubricate your skin and acts as a waterproof shield. Sweat glands also help to protect your skin. This layer also contains your hair follicles.

Subcutaneous fat: This layer of skin is mainly made up of fat and is responsible for keeping the body warm. It also helps to act as a shock absorber, when you bang into something or fall, it will help to cushion the blow.

Here is a list of some of the functions that your skin performs:

- It helps to diminish the harmful affects of UV rays of the sun.
- It acts as a protective barrier against any kind of hazardous substance or injury.
- It prevents loss of moisture.
- It is a sensory organ that can detect temperature and touch.
- It aids in the regulation of temperature.
- It is an immune organ that can detect infections within the body.
- It helps to manufacture vitamin D.

It is impressive that this one organ has so many functions. There is surely more to our skin than meets the eye. I would think that such an important organ deserves some exceptional care and attention.

The cosmetic and beauty industry is one that is thriving, with many individuals spending in the upwards of hundreds of dollars a month to look beautiful. People should spend more time researching and understanding more about the skin products that they are using and spending their money on. By understanding the needs or requirements of your skin you will be better able to provide it with the proper nourishment that it needs.

To be able to provide your skin with the right products, you need to be aware of the type of skin that you have. There are many factors that skin types are based around; such as water content in your skin (this has an impact on your skin's elasticity. The amount of oil in your skin has an impact on your skin's softness and the sensitivity levels of your skin.

There are four skin types that your skin may be classified into:

1. Oily skin

2. Dry skin

3. Normal skin

4. Combination skin

Dry skin: The medical term used to describe dry skin is xeroderma. You might have dry skin if you feel tightness right after you have washed your skin. Your skin has very little to no shine to it, it looks dull. It can produce a rough complexion, visible lines, red patches, less elasticity, and almost invisible pores.

If dry skin is exposed to drying factors, this can lead to cracked and peeling skin, that can become inflamed and itchy. If your skin appears scaly and rough, then it is very dry. Factors that can lead to dry skin include:

- Weather conditions (such as wind, sun or extreme cold).
- Genetics
- Aging
- Hormonal changes
- Excessive indoor heating
- Medications
- Certain soaps and cosmetics
- Hot showers
- UV radiations from tanning beds

Oily skin: Your skin produces some natural oils. Now, some individuals will produce more oils than others. This can lead to oily skin. Oily skin can cause you to have a thick complexion that may appear dull or shiny. Oily skin can cause enlarged pores, pimples, blemishes and blackheads. Some factors that may lead to oily skin are the following:

- Puberty
- Hormonal imbalances
- Excessive exposure to humidity or heat
- Stress

Normal skin: Normal skin is skin that is neither too dry nor too oily. Normal skin demonstrates it presence by a few imperfections, barely visible pores, radiant skin complexion and no skin sensitivity.

Combination skin: Combination skin is a very common kind of skin type. It appears as normal or dry in some areas and oily in other areas. Usually the T-zone or nose area is where it is oily, along with the forehead and chin areas. People that have combination skin will often have dilated pores, shiny skin and blackheads.

Now that you have a better understanding of your skin type this will help you to decide the skin care products that will best suit your personal needs. The basic need of your skin, regardless of skin type is hydration. There are two kinds of hydration elements:

- *The humectants:* these are the ones that will help to preserve moisture.
- *The lubricants:* lubricants help to form a protective layer on your skin. This does not allow the moisture to leave your skin.

Caring for Your Skin

In our everyday life, we are constantly surrounded with toxins and pollutants. These things affect our health, including the health of our skin. Toxins cause our skin to age faster. Our skin battles constantly trying to protect us from viruses, germs, bacteria and toxins lurking outside of our bodies. The more that we subject our skin to these poisons, the more our skin ages. Have you ever really read the labels of the products that you are putting on your skin? Unless you are using products that are 100% organic, there is a high chance you are using something that is doing more harm then good. The central premises to 'clean living' is in the removing of harmful chemicals from our lives. You not only want to eat clean foods, but you should also want to use clean and healthy ingredients on your skin.

The movement for clean living is growing, more and more organic products are being sold. Many stores are adding organic selections in foods and other products. This movement is fighting against genetically modified organisms (GMO) in our foods. A huge step in healthier living is utilizing organic products.

So, how can we take care of this large organ, known quite simply as 'skin'? There are several common-sense things that we can do to help keep our skin healthy.

- **Nutrition:** Eating a healthy diet will indeed help to benefit your skin.
- **Hydration:** Keeping your skin hydrated by drinking plenty of water, will help it to get rid of impurities.
- **Sleep:** During sleep our skin works hard at repairing itself. It is during this time that Collagen production is at its highest.
- **Cleansing:** Throughout the day our skin is constantly under attack from all kinds of pollutants and impurities. Be good to your skin by cleansing it regularly.
- **Don't smoke:** The impurities and pollutants in cigarettes will cause your skin to age faster.
- **Sunscreen:** Protect your skin from the harmful rays of the sun. Use sunscreen if you are out in the hottest part of the day.

Chapter 2. Making Homemade Body Butters

The wonderful thing about making your own homemade body butters is that basic body butters can be made with just one or two ingredients. You will find these ingredients in your house or at your local supermarket. Some of the basic butters you can use are Shea butter, mango butter, cocoa butter just to name a few. Below are some easy to prepare body butter recipes that I am sure you are going to love!

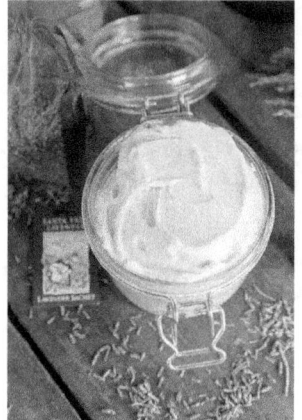

1. Lavender Body Butter
This body butter is calming, relaxing and rejuvenating. This will help to treat sunburn, with its great nourishing and cooling affects.

Ingredients:

- ¼ cup honey
- ½ cup beeswax
- 1 cup coconut oil
- 4 tablespoons Aloe Vera gel
- 20 drops lavender essential oil
- 1 vitamin E capsule
- ¼ cup olive oil
- 2 tablespoons Lanolin

Directions:

In a saucepan melt the olive oil, coconut oil, beeswax, and honey over low heat, using a double broiler method. Using the same double broiler method in a separate pan heat the Aloe Vera and then mix it with beeswax mix until it is melted. Continue to stir. Add in the lanolin and continue to gently stir. Remove from heat and add in the lavender essential oil and the vitamin E. Whip mixture with hand blender until it is light and fluffy. Pour it into a glass jar and allow it to cool before using.

2. Mango Body Butter

Mango butter contains elevated levels of antioxidants that help to facilitate clearing and softening of skin, helping to eliminate blemishes and blackheads while cleaning clogged pores. It helps to cool your body and leave a healthy glow to your skin. The lovely fruity aroma of this body butter will have you wanting to use it again and again.

Ingredients:

- 1 cup coconut oil
- ½ cup Shea butter
- ½ cup Mango butter
- 30 drops mango essential oil

Directions:

In a saucepan melt the Shea butter, coconut oil together over low heat, using a double broiler method. Slowly stir and add in the mango butter. Remove from heat and allow it to cool for a few minutes. Add in the mango essential oil. Whip the mixture until it becomes light and fluffy. Place into glass container. Allow it to sit at room temperature overnight to harden.

3. Magnesium Body Butter

Magnesium is a wonderful thing that helps with the absorption of vitamin D. It works wonders on sore muscles and safely used on children owing to its all natural ingredients. It will help to nourish your skin making it soft and silky!

Ingredients:

- 4 tablespoons of beeswax
- ½ cup coconut oil
- ¼ cup Shea butter
- ½ cup of natural magnesium flakes

Directions:

In a mixing bowl add in the magnesium flakes, then pour three tablespoons of boiling water over them. Stir them until they dissolve and a thick liquid has formed. Set aside to cool. Using the double broiler method, take the Shea butter, beeswax, and coconut oil and add to a pan. Place over low heat until they melt and blend together. Once they have blended, remove them from the heat and allow to cool. Pour the magnesium into this mixture when it has cooled. Whip mix with hand blender. Whip for about ten minutes and then store mix in the fridge. When mix achieves a semi solid consistency whip it again. Pour into a glass container, seal it with lid and store it in a cool, dry place. You can keep a small batch of this mix up to three months.

4. Sweet Orange Body Butter

The lovely aroma of orange and lemon combined is so very refreshing—it will have you feeling awake in no time while filling you with energy. Use this mixture after a morning shower to get that extra boost of energy to help give you that kick start to your morning.

Ingredients:

- ½ cup sweet almond oil
- 1 cup Shea butter
- ½ cup coconut oil
- 20 drops sweet orange essential oil
- 10 drops lemon essential oil

Directions:

Using the double broiler method melt the Shea butter in a pan. Now add in the coconut oil and stir to blend. Remove from heat and place mixture at room temperature for thirty minutes. Add the sweet almond oil, lemon essential oil and sweet orange essential oil to mix once it has cooled down. Stir the mixture and then place it into the fridge for two hours. Once it has achieved a semi solid consistency whip it with a hand blender until it forms peaks. Transfer mixture into glass jar and seal with lid, storing in cool, dry place.

5. Peppermint Body Butter

Peppermint body butter is easy to prepare, offering a divine smelling body butter. It works great for sore muscles, cramps and is a wonderful way to nourish your dry winter skin.

Ingredients:

- ½ cup Shea butter
- ½ cup coconut oil
- ½ cup cocoa butter
- ½ cup sweet almond oil
- 6 drops peppermint essential oil
- 12 drops vitamin E extract

Directions:

Using the double broiler method, melt cocoa butter, Shea butter, and coconut oil. Remove from heat and allow to cool at room temperature. Once mix has cooled add in peppermint essential oil and vitamin E extract and mix well. Keep mix in your fridge for two hours, or until it contains a semi solid consistency. Whip mix with your hand blender until it forms peaks. Add mix into glass container, and seal with lid, storing it in a cool, dry place.

Chapter 3. Homemade Lotion Recipes

This collection of homemade lotion recipes offers a variety of health benefits!

6. Simple Sunscreen Baby Lotion

This lotion will offer an overall moisturizing lotion with added protection against the harmful effects of the sun.

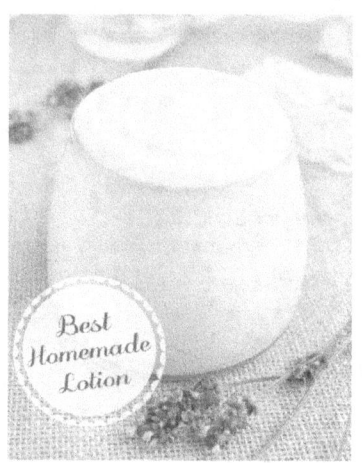

Ingredients:

- 4-6 sprays of sunscreen
- 8 ounces Vaseline
- 16 ounces baby oil

Directions:

Put all your ingredients into a mixing bowl. Mix ingredients using a whisk. Add mixture to glass jar and use as required.

7. Lavender Body Lotion

This lotion will help to treat Eczema, as coconut oil is beneficial in treating eczema. When combined with the lavender it offers a calming, soothing and repairing benefit for your skin.

Ingredients:

- 2 tablespoons of beeswax
- 1/3 cup coconut oil

- 7 drops lavender essential oil

Directions:

Heat up some water over low heat. Place coconut oil and beeswax into a glass jar. Add in the heated water, allowing the beeswax to completely melt. Allow the mixture to cool. Add in the lavender essential oil. Using your hand blender, blend mixture until it resembles a soft lotion. Store in a glass jar, seal with lid, store in a cool, dry place.

8. Rose Lotion

Rose lotion works great at helping to relieve anxiety and everyday life stresses. The 'rose' in the lotion helps to act as a 'balancer' to place you in a more relaxed state of mind.

Ingredients:

- ¼ cup extra virgin olive oil
- ¼ cup coconut oil
- ¾ cup rose water
- 2 ¼ tablespoons grated beeswax
- 10 drops rose essential oil

Directions:

Heat some water in a pan over low heat. Add in beeswax, and allow it to melt, stir often for about 20 minutes. Remove from heat and allow to cool at room temperature. Blend with hand blender, until desired consistency is reached. Allow to sit for 5 minutes, then place in the rose essential oil. Store lotion in a glass jar, seal with lid, and store in a cool, dry place.

9. Vanilla Body Lotion

All three oils in this lotion are natural skin moisturizers and the vanilla has natural sugars which help to retain your skin moisture. It also serves as a protective barrier on your skin. If your skin is dry this lotion will provide it with the boost it needs.

Ingredients:

- 1 vanilla pod
- ½ cup Jojoba oil
- ½ cup almond oil
- 1 cup cocoa butter

Directions:

Melt the jojoba oil and cocoa butter over low heat until the two have melted together. Remove from heat and allow to cool for 30 minutes. Place mix in a mixing bowl. Slit the vanilla pod and scrape the inside of it into the bowl. Add the almond oil and mix well. Add to a container that you can place in your freezer. Allow it to solidify in freezer for 30 minutes. Remove mix from freezer and using your hand mixer whip it until you get desired consistency. Add lotion to glass jar, sealing with lid, and storing in cool, dry place.

10. Aloe Body Lotion

This lotion works great on sunburnt and sensitive skin. This lotion works wonders at replenishing skin cells. Aloe is high in anti-oxidants properties which help to promote skin healing.

Ingredients:

- ½ cup almond oil
- ½ cup Aloe Vera gel

Directions:

Mix your almond oil and Aloe Vera gel in a mixing bowl. Add mixture to a glass jar, seal with lid and store in a cool, dry place. Use this lotion after you have come out of the sun.

Chapter 4. Homemade Balm Recipes

Certain times of the year dry out your lips, especially during the winter season, and during changes of seasons. None of us like to have chapped lips, causing our lips to become dry and sensitive. When choosing a lip balm, you should make sure that you are aware of the ingredients in it, especially since we ingest whatever is on our lips. Using food-based ingredients, will help to ensure that it is safe to ingest.

11. Chocolate Lip Balm

You are probably surprised to hear that dark chocolate is good for your skin. It offers anti-inflammatory and anti-oxidant properties. It also offers sun protection qualities that will shield your skin from the damaging UV rays. Cocoa butter is also good at helping to lower bad cholesterol, and is a great moisturizer for your skin.

Ingredients:

- 1 teaspoon cocoa butter
- 1 teaspoon beeswax
- 1 teaspoon sweet almond oil
- 6 dark chocolate chips
- 1 capsule of vitamin E

Directions:

Using the double broiler method, heat the cocoa butter, and almond oil over low heat, just enough to melt them together. Remove from heat and allow to cool, add in remaining ingredients. Use an eyedropper to transfer mixture to container.

12. Lemongrass Lip Balm

Lemongrass essential oil offers a strong lineup for minerals and vitamins: copper, calcium, iron, folate, magnesium, potassium, manganese, vitamins B1, B2, B3, B6, C, and zinc. It also offers antibacterial, antioxidant, antifungal, and anti-inflammatory properties, while helping to promote feelings of tranquility and peace.

Ingredients:

- 1 tablespoon beeswax
- 1 tablespoon coconut oil
- ½ teaspoon vitamin E oil
- 10 drops lemongrass essential oil

Directions:

Using the double broiler method, melt the coconut oil and beeswax over low heat until melted. Remove from heat and add in vitamin E oil and lemongrass essential oil. Mix and pour into container, sealing with lid, store in a cool, dry place.

13. Vanilla Lip Balm

Vanilla essential oil with it's sweet aroma offers a very calming and relaxing feeling. When you use it in your lip balm that it right under your nose it will work great as a form of aromatherapy. Honey offers strong antioxidants, antibacterial, anti-aging properties. It is also soothing and moisturizing, and works well in lip balms.

Ingredients:

- ¼ ounce beeswax

- 1 teaspoon organic honey
- 10 drops vanilla essential oil
- 2 ounces sweet almond oil

Directions:

Using the double broiler method, heat the beeswax and almond oil until they are melted. Remove from heat and allow to cool, add in the remaining ingredients. Transfer mixture into glass jar, seal with lid and store in a cool, dry place.

14. Peppermint Lip Balm

The peppermint essential oil will offer a great calming effect, working as an aromatherapy treatment as your nose will smell the aroma of this lip balm, bringing peace and calm to you.

Ingredients:

- 2 ounces of grapeseed oil
- 10 drops of peppermint essential oil
- ¼ ounce of beeswax
- 1 teaspoon organic honey

Directions:

Using the broiler method, heat the beeswax and grapeseed oil over low heat until melted. Once melted remove from heat and allow to cool for a few minutes. Add in the remaining ingredients and mix well. Add to glass jar, seal with lid and store in cool, dry place.

15. Mango Lip Balm
Ingredients:

- 10 drops mango essential oil
- 2 ounces grapeseed oil
- 1 teaspoon organic honey
- ¼ ounce of beeswax

Directions:

Using the broiler method, melt the beeswax and grapeseed oil over low heat. Once melted remove from heat and add in the remaining ingredients. Add to glass jar, seal with lid and store in cool, dry place.

Chapter 5. Homemade Bath Bomb Recipes

After you have had a long stressful day there is nothing like going home to soak in your bath tub to wash all the stress of the day away. You can create your own home spa with a few candles, a glass of wine and homemade bath bombs.   Using these bath bombs as a form of aromatherapy will help you to enjoy this at home spa experience with the relaxing effect they will have over you.

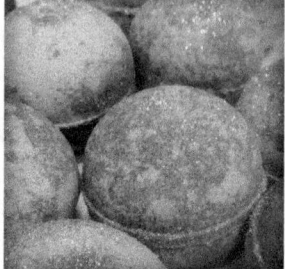

16. Green Tea Bath Bomb
Green tea is great for you both inside and out. It offers antibacterial and anti-inflammatory properties. It also helps to fight against aging skin. The tannins in the tea will shrink pores and work well for treating oily skin.

Ingredients:

- ½ cup citric acid
- 1 ¼ cups baking soda
- 2 teaspoons sweet almond oil
- ½ tablespoon water
- 5 drops of green food coloring
- 2 tablespoons of green tea leaves

Directions:

Combine all your dry ingredients, except for the tea leaves. Mix the almond oil, and food coloring and drizzle this over dry ingredient. Mix well using your hands. Add half a tablespoon of boiling water to the tea leaves. Add them to mixture. Press lightly into oiled molds. Remove from molds and let them dry.

17. Bubbly Milk Bath

Baking soda offers both microbial and alkaline properties. It will sooth your skin and help with irritated skin, insect bites, rashes and acne. It will also help to exfoliate dead skin cells. The lemon essential oil offers many benefits for your skin. It is an astringent and antiseptic and will help to rejuvenate your skin bringing back a bright luster to it.

Ingredients:

- ½ cup citric acid
- 1 cup baking soda
- ½ cup corn starch
- ¼ cup powdered milk
- 1/3 cup Epsom salts, finely ground
- 2 tablespoons olive oil
- 1 teaspoon lemon essential oil
- 2 teaspoons melted cocoa butter
- 7 teaspoons distilled water

Directions:

Using the double broiler method, heat cocoa butter, olive oil until melted over low heat. Mix the dry ingredients in a bowl. Drizzle the cocoa butter mix over the dry ingredients. Add in the lemon essential oil. Spray with water to bring to right consistency. Add to molds. Set aside and allow them to dry.

18. Lavender Bath Bomb

Citric acid offers several benefits for your skin. It can help to unclog your pores. It also offers anti-aging properties and is loaded with antioxidants. It also contains an alpha-hydroxy acid which helps to exfoliate dead skin cells

Ingredients:

- 1 cup baking soda

- 1 teaspoon water
- 2 teaspoons lavender essential oil
- ½ cup Epsom salts
- ½ cup citric acid
- 3 teaspoons olive oil
- 3 drops of food coloring of your choice

Directions:

Mix your dry ingredients in a large mixing bowl. Combine your wet ingredients in a small bowl. Pour a small amount of your wet mix into the dry mix and whisk. Add another small amount and whisk again, continuing to do this until the process is complete. Add mix into molds. Remove from molds and allow bath bombs to dry.

19. Vanilla Bath Bomb
Enjoy a lovely soak in a tub while you get some aromatherapy smelling the wonderful aroma of the vanilla in your bath bomb that will have you feeling relaxed and come in no time!

Ingredients:

- 10 drops vanilla essential oil
- ½ cup citric acid
- 1 cup baking soda
- 1 teaspoon water
- 3 teaspoons almond oil
- ½ cup Epsom salts, finely ground
- 3 drops yellow food coloring

Directions:

Mix your dry ingredients in a large mixing bowl. Combine your wet ingredients in a small bowl. Pour a small amount of your wet mix into the dry mix and whisk. Add another small amount and whisk again, continuing to do this until the process is complete. Add mix into molds. Remove from molds and allow bath bombs to dry.

20. Rose Bath Bomb

The rose essential oil will work as a form of aromatherapy, helping you to sink into your tub and relax, melting away the stresses of the day.

Ingredients:

- 10 drops rose essential oil
- 1 teaspoon of rose water
- ½ cup citric acid
- 1 cup baking soda
- 3 teaspoons olive oil
- ½ cup Epsom salts, finely ground
- 3 drops of food coloring of your choice

Directions:

Mix your dry ingredients in a large mixing bowl. Combine your wet ingredients in a small bowl. Pour a small amount of your wet mix into the dry mix and whisk. Add another small amount and whisk again, continuing to do this until the process is complete. Add mix into molds. Remove from molds and allow bath bombs to dry.

Chapter 6. Homemade Scrubs

Here are some wonderful recipes for salt and sugar scrubs, both of which work as exfoliants. The purpose behind exfoliants is to remove dead skin cells. There are also several other benefits to scrubs: improved circulation, reduction in cellulite, and anti-aging just to name a few. Treating your body to a scrub will help you to relax during this treatment that is healthy and beneficial to you.

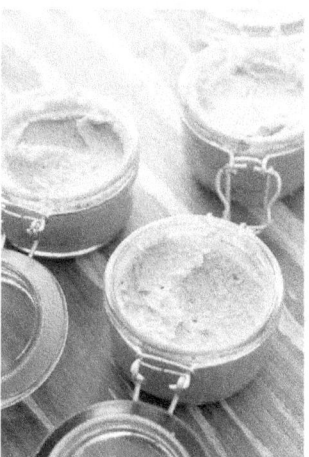

21. Mocha Salt Scrub
If you love the smell of chocolate and coffee, then this could easily become your favorite salt scrub.

Ingredients:

- ½ cup nourishing oil
- ¾ cup sea salt
- ¼ cup unsweetened cocoa or freeze-dried coffee
- 1 teaspoon vanilla extract
- 2 tablespoons of organic honey

Directions:

Mix all the ingredients together, then add them to a glass jar and store in a cool, dry place.

22. Citrus Salt Scrub

Citrus is great to use to help moisturize your skin, it is also a great toner. It is good for you both inside and out.

Ingredients:

- ½ cup nourishing oil
- ½ cup sea salt
- ½ teaspoon lemon zest
- ½ teaspoon orange zest

Directions:

Mix all the ingredients together, then add them to a glass jar and store in a cool, dry place.

23. Clean Face Scrub
Ingredients:

- Virgin olive oil
- Sea salt

Directions:

Mix equal portions of both virgin olive oil and sea salt. Store in glass jar, in cool, dry place.

24. Lavender Scrub

Lavender essential oil has many benefits, but one of the most well-known is its calming effects. You can help get rid of your daily stresses in life when you use this lavender scrub. It will help to lift your spirits and having you feeling uplifted in no time!

Ingredients:

- 1 cup sea salt (Himalayan pink sea salt has 84 trace minerals that would be great for your skin).
- 10 drops lavender essential oil
- ½ cup nourishing oil such as almond oil or grapeseed oil
- Dried lavender (optional)

Directions:

Mix all the ingredients together, then add them to a glass jar and store in a cool, dry place.

25. Peppermint Scrub
Ingredients:

- 10 drops peppermint essential oil
- 1 cup sea salt, Himalayan pink sea salt would be best to use on skin.
- ½ cup avocado oil

Directions:

Mix all the ingredients together, then add them to a glass jar and store in a cool, dry place.

Conclusion

I hope that you and your loved ones will enjoy using these natural and healthy skin care recipes that are easy to prepare, and will have awesome results! If you want to live a healthier and clean lifestyle keeping yourself healthy inside and out will give you that overall health and well-being you are searching for. This collection of skin care natural recipes will cover the outside part of keeping your skin healthy!

I would like to thank you once again for downloading my book, your support of my work means a great deal to me. I would love to read a review of my book by you on Amazon!

FREE Bonus Reminder

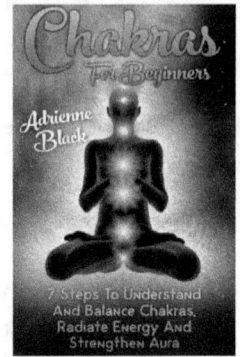

If you have not grabbed it yet, please go ahead and download your special bonus E book *"Chakras for Beginners. 7 Steps To Understand And Balance Chakras, Radiate Energy, And Strengthen Aura"*.

Simply Click the Button Below

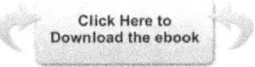

OR **Go to This Page**

http://lifehacksworld.com/free

BONUS #2: More Free Books

Do you want to receive more Free Books?

We have a mailing list where we send out our new Books when they go free on Kindle. Click on the link below to sign up for Free Book Promotions.

=> Sign Up for Free Book Promotions <=

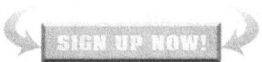

OR Go to this URL

http://zbit.ly/1WBb1Ek